The

COMPLETE KEGEL EXERCISES

for Men

The Detailed Practical Guide to Treat Premature Ejaculation, Sexual and Erectile Dysfunction | Improve Male Reproductive Health System

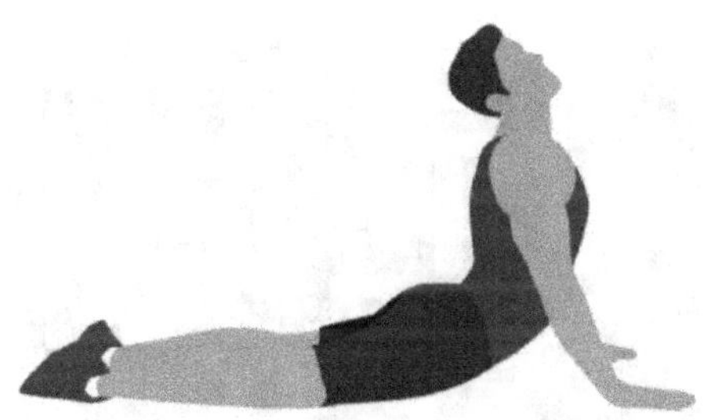

ERIC A. RANDELL

ERIC A. RANDELL

COPYRIGHT

GAIN ACCESS TO MORE BOOKS FROM ME

TABLE OF CONTENTS

INTRODUCTION

As men, we often overlook the importance of maintaining our pelvic floor muscles. However, taking care of our pelvic health is essential for various aspects of our well-being, especially when it comes to sexual and reproductive health. Kegel exercises offer a simple and effective way to enhance pelvic floor strength, addressing common issues like erectile dysfunction, premature ejaculation, low sperm count, and overall reproductive health.

For many men, struggling with erectile dysfunction can be incredibly disheartening. The good news is that Kegel exercises can significantly improve erectile function by strengthening the muscles responsible for sustaining an erection. By incorporating a regular Kegel exercise routine, many men have found that they experience better blood flow to the pelvic area and improved control over their erections, thereby boosting their confidence and satisfaction with their sexual performance.

Moreover, Kegel exercises can help men last longer in bed by enhancing the endurance and control of their pelvic floor muscles. This can lead to increased pleasure and satisfaction for both themselves and their partners, ultimately enriching the overall sexual experience.

In addition to addressing sexual health issues, Kegel exercises have proven to positively impact reproductive health. Low sperm count can be a significant concern for men who are hoping to start a family, but studies have indicated that Kegel exercises contribute to increased sperm production and motility, which can ultimately improve fertility.

Throughout this book, we will delve into the science behind Kegel exercises for men, exploring various techniques, benefits, and practical applications to improve pelvic floor health. By understanding and incorporating Kegel exercises, men can take proactive steps to boost their sexual performance, tackle reproductive challenges, and overall improve their quality of life. Let's embark on this journey to reclaim and optimize our pelvic floor health, leading to greater physical and sexual well-being. For cookbook filled with delicious recipes to boost male sexual fertility, click here.

Benefits of Kegel Exercises to Men

Kegel exercises can be incredibly beneficial for men in several ways. Here are some of the top reasons why Kegel exercises are important to men especially:

1. Improved Erectile Function: Kegel exercises can help strengthen the pelvic floor muscles, which play a crucial role in sustaining an erection. By regularly practicing Kegel exercises, men can enhance the blood flow to the pelvic region, which can lead to improved erectile function and overall sexual performance.

2. Addressing Premature Ejaculation: Strong pelvic floor muscles can contribute to better control over ejaculation, allowing men to improve their stamina and endurance during sexual activity. Both couples may be more satisfied as a result of this.

3. **Urinary Incontinence:** Kegel exercises can be beneficial for men who experience issues with urinary incontinence. By strengthening the pelvic floor muscles, men can achieve better control over their bladder, reducing instances of leakage.

4. **Pelvic Health:** Maintaining a healthy pelvic floor is essential for overall physical well-being. Strong pelvic floor muscles can support the organs in the pelvic region, contributing to better posture, core strength, and lower back health.

5. **Reproductive Health:** Kegel exercises have also been linked to improved reproductive health in men. They can help increase sperm production and motility, potentially aiding in fertility for men who are trying to start a family.

Some FAQs About Kegel Exercises for Men

Q: What are Kegel exercises for men and why are they important?

A: Kegel exercises for men involve the contraction and relaxation of the pelvic floor muscles, which are essential for bladder control, sexual function, and overall pelvic health. Strengthening these muscles through Kegel exercises can help improve urinary incontinence, enhance erectile function, and promote overall pelvic floor health.

Q: How do I locate my pelvic floor muscles to perform Kegel exercises?

A: To identify your pelvic floor muscles, try stopping the flow of urine mid-stream. The muscles used to do this are the same ones targeted in Kegel exercises. However, it's important to note that this should only be done for the purpose of identifying the muscles, and not as a regular practice.

Q: Can Kegel exercise help with premature ejaculation?

A: Yes, Kegel exercises can contribute to better control over ejaculation, potentially helping to address premature ejaculation. By strengthening the pelvic floor muscles, men may experience increased stamina and improved control during sexual activity.

Q: How long does it take to see the benefits of Kegel exercises?

A: The timeline for experiencing the benefits of Kegel exercises can vary from person to person. Some men may notice improvements within a few weeks, while for others, it may take longer. Consistency and regular practice are key to seeing results.

Q: How often should I perform Kegel exercises?

A: It's recommended to perform Kegel exercises at least three times a day, aiming for about 10-15 repetitions during each session. Over time, as the muscles become stronger, the number of repetitions can be increased.

Q: Can Kegel exercises improve sexual performance and satisfaction?

A: Yes, strengthening the pelvic floor muscles through Kegel exercises can lead to improved erectile function, better control over ejaculation, and enhanced sexual stamina. All of these factors can contribute to increased sexual satisfaction for both men and their partners.

Q: Are there any risks or side effects associated with Kegel exercises for men?

A: When performed correctly, Kegel exercises are generally safe and pose minimal risks. However, it's important to avoid overdoing the exercises, as this could lead to muscle fatigue or strain. If you have any concerns or experience discomfort while performing Kegel exercises, it's advisable to consult a healthcare professional.

Items Needed for Kegel Exercise

- ✓ Kegel balls or weights
- ✓ Exercise mat
- ✓ Comfortable clothing
- ✓ A chair or exercise bench
- ✓ Lubricant (optional)
- ✓ Timer or stopwatch (optional)
- ✓ Towel (optional)

Instructions for Kegel Exercises

- ✓ **Find a comfortable position:** Sit, stand, or lie down in a comfortable position. It's important to be relaxed when doing Kegel exercises.

- ✓ **Identify the right muscles:** The first step is to correctly identify the pelvic floor muscles. These are the muscles used to stop the flow of urine or prevent passing gas. To do this, imagine you are trying to stop the flow of urine or tighten the muscles that keep you from passing gas. These are the muscles you should focus on when doing Kegel exercises.

✓ **Start with contraction:** Once you have identified the right muscles, begin the exercise by contracting or squeezing those muscles. It's important not to tense the muscles in the abdomen, thighs, or buttocks. Make sure to concentrate on the pelvic floor muscles.

✓ **Hold the contraction:** Hold the contraction for 3-5 seconds. It is important to breathe normally and avoid holding your breath during the exercise.

✓ **Relax the muscles:** After holding the contraction, relax the pelvic floor muscles for an equal amount of time or 3-5 seconds. This completes one repetition.

✓ **Repeat the exercise:** Aim to complete a set of 10-15 repetitions. As your muscles strengthen, gradually increase the number of repetitions.

✓ **Aim for consistency:** It's important to integrate Kegel exercises into your daily routine. Start with one set of 10-15 repetitions and gradually work up to

3-4 sets per day. Consistency is key to seeing improvements in reproductive health.

Kegel exercises can be performed discreetly and at any time throughout the day, making them an easily accessible exercise for men seeking to improve their reproductive health. As with any exercise program, it is recommended to consult with a healthcare professional before beginning, especially if there are any underlying health concerns.

LET US BEGIN THE JOURNEY

The Cat-Cow Stretch

The Cat-Cow stretch is a yoga pose that helps to improve flexibility and mobility of the spine, while also supporting pelvic floor health.

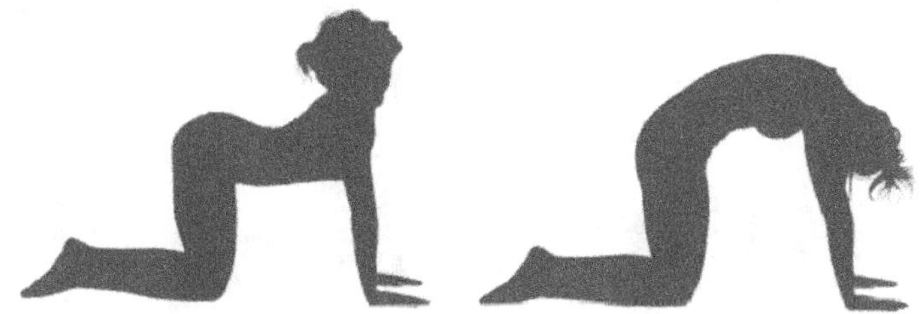

Instructions:

- ✓ Start on your hands and knees, align your wrists under your shoulders and your knees under your hips. Spread your fingers wide for stability.

- ✓ Inhale as you arch your back, dropping your belly toward the floor, and lifting your head and tailbone towards the ceiling. This is the "Cow" position. Hold for 5-10 seconds, breathing deeply and allowing your belly to drop towards the floor.

- ✓ As you exhale, round your spine up towards the ceiling, tucking your chin to your chest and pulling your belly button in towards your spine. This is the "Cat" position. Hold for 5-10 seconds, feeling the stretch through your back.

✓ Continue to move between the Cat and Cow positions, syncing your breath with the movement. Breathe in air as you move into a Cow and breathe out air as you move into a Cat.

Elevated Glute Bridge

Elevated glute bridge is an effective exercise to strengthen the glutes, hamstrings, and pelvic floor muscles.

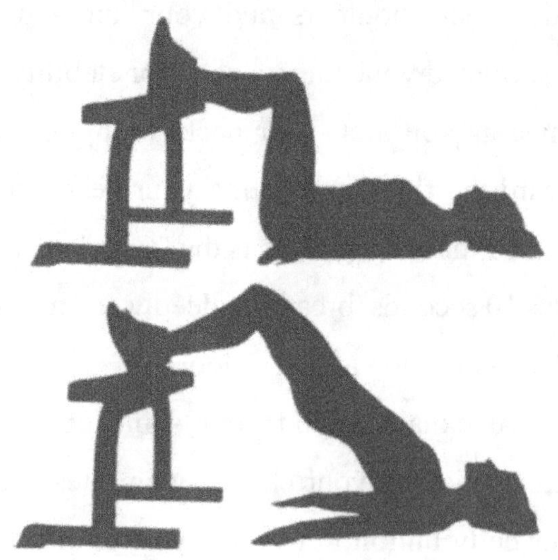

Instructions:

- ✓ Lie on your back, knees bending, feet flat on the floor. Place your heels on a raised surface such as a bench, step, or sturdy box.
- ✓ Engage your core and buttocks as you lift your hips upward towards the ceiling. At the height of the action, your body should create a straight line from your shoulders to your knees.
- ✓ Hold the position for 3-5 seconds, focusing on squeezing your glutes and pelvic floor muscles.
- ✓ Slowly and carefully lower your hips back to the starting position.
- ✓ Aim to complete 10-15 repetitions of the elevated glute bridge.

Lying Hip Abduction

Lying hip abduction is a beneficial exercise for improving hip and pelvic muscle strength.

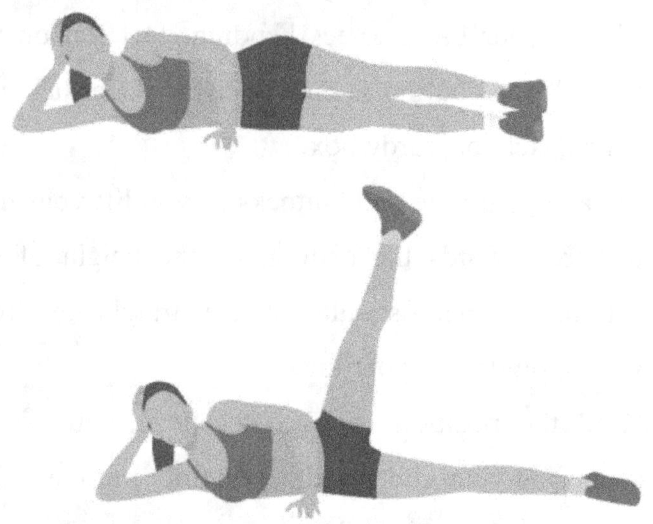

Instructions:

- ✓ Begin by lying on one side on a comfortable surface, such as a yoga mat.

- ✓ Rest your head on your lower arm for support and place your upper hand on the ground in front of you to maintain balance.

- ✓ Keep your lower leg straight and slightly bend your upper leg for stability.

- ✓ Slowly raise your upper leg toward the ceiling, keeping the foot flexed and the leg straight. Be sure to engage your outer hip muscles as you perform the movement.

- ✓ Hold the raised position for 2-3 seconds to maximize muscle engagement.
- ✓ Gently lower your leg back to the starting position to complete one repetition.
- ✓ Aim to perform 10-15 repetitions on each leg, then switch to work the opposite side.

Seated Pelvic Tilt

Seated pelvic tilt is an excellent Kegel exercise that can help improve reproductive health in men.

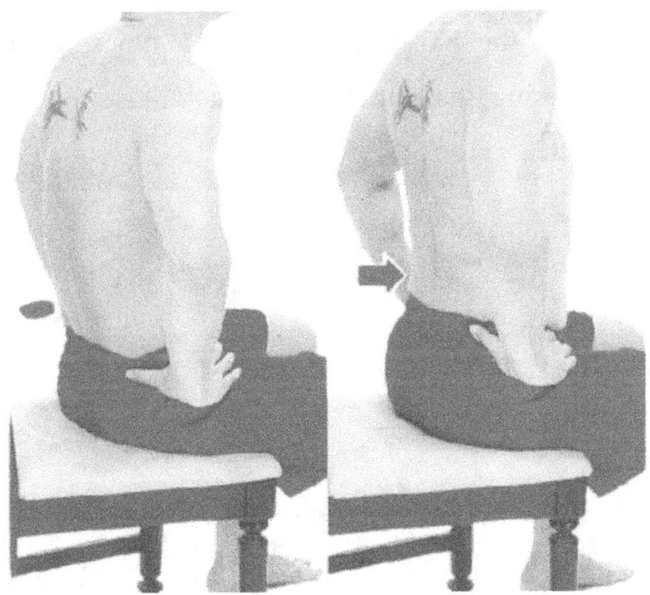

Instructions:

- ✓ Sit on the floor (or any flat surface) with your legs extended in front of you.

- ✓ Place your hands on the floor beside your hips for support.

- ✓ Take a deep breath in and as you exhale, tilt your pelvis forward by engaging your pelvic floor muscles.

- ✓ Hold the tilt for 5-10 seconds while continuing to breathe normally.

- ✓ Release the tilt and return to the starting position.

- ✓ Repeat the movement for 10-15 times, gradually increasing the number as you build strength and control.

The Leg Slide

The leg slide exercise is a Kegel exercise that can help improve reproductive health in men.

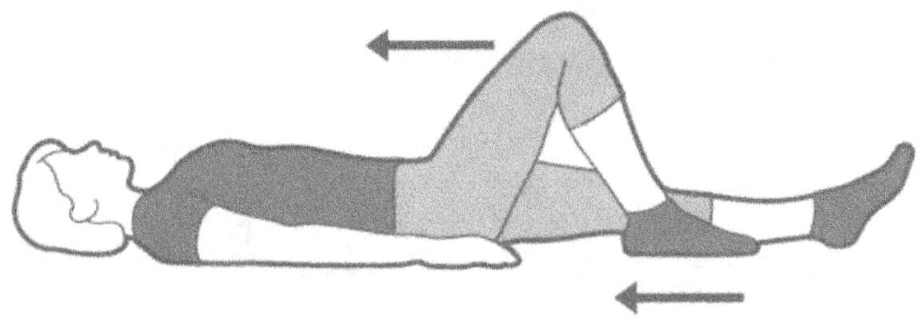

Instructions:

- ✓ Lie down on your back on a flat surface, such as a yoga mat or bed.
- ✓ Bend your knees, keeping your feet flat on the surface and hip-width apart.
- ✓ Engage your pelvic floor muscles by imagining that you are stopping the flow of urine mid-stream.
- ✓ Slowly slide one foot away from your body, straightening your leg along the surface while keeping your pelvic floor engaged. It's important to keep the movement controlled and avoid using the leg muscles to slide the foot.

- ✓ Hold the extended position for 5-10 seconds, continuing to engage the pelvic floor muscles.
- ✓ Slowly slide the foot back to the starting position, maintaining the engagement of the pelvic floor muscles throughout the movement.
- ✓ Repeat the same movement with the other leg.

Hip Flexor Stretch

Hip flexor stretch is a great exercise to improve flexibility and mobility in the hips, which can have a positive impact on overall reproductive health.

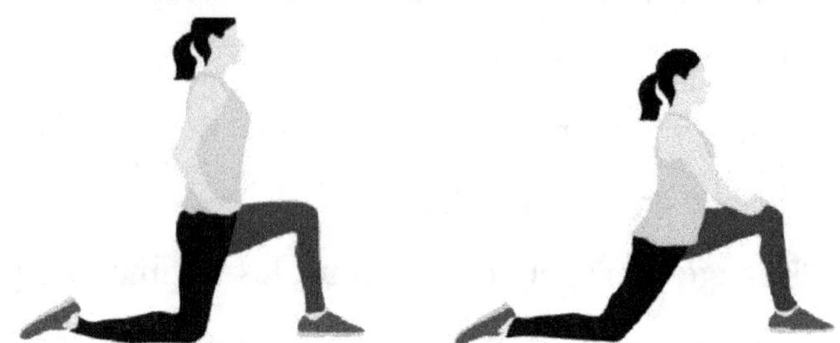

Instructions:

- ✓ Begin in a kneeling position on the floor with one knee bent at a 90-degree angle in front of you and the other leg extended behind you.

- ✓ Keeping your upper body straight, gently shift your weight forward, leaning into the front knee until you feel a stretch in the hip of the extended leg.
- ✓ Hold this position for 30 seconds to 1 minute, focusing on breathing deeply and relaxing into the stretch.
- ✓ Repeat the stretch on the other side by switching the position of your legs.
- ✓ Aim to perform 2-3 sets of the stretch on each side.

The Frog Pose

The frog pose is an effective yoga pose that can help stretch the inner thighs and groin area, improving flexibility and mobility in the hip region.

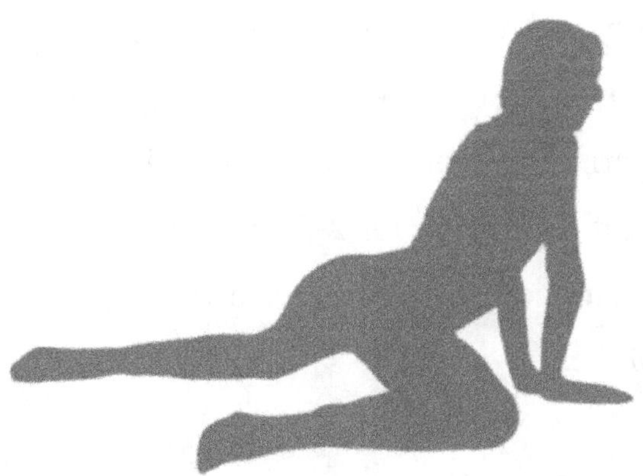

Instructions:

- ✓ Start by coming down to the floor on your hands and knees, with your hands directly below your shoulders and your knees directly below your hips.

- ✓ Slowly begin to slide your knees apart as wide as you comfortably can, keeping your ankles in line with your knees.

- ✓ Flex your feet so that the inner arches of your feet are flat on the floor, and your toes are pointing slightly outward.

- ✓ Lower your hips towards the ground, feeling a deep stretch in your inner thighs and groin area. You can also lower down onto your forearms for a deeper stretch.

- ✓ Hold the pose for 30 seconds to 1 minute, breathing deeply and relaxing into the stretch.

- ✓ Slowly release the pose by pressing into your hands and bringing your knees back together.

- ✓ Repeat the stretch for 2-3 sets, gradually increasing the duration of the stretch as your flexibility improves.

Standing Pelvic Tilt

Standing pelvic tilt is a Kegel exercise that can help improve reproductive health for men.

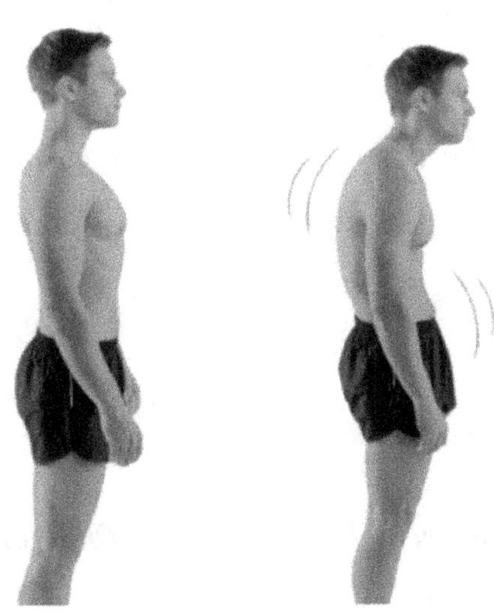

Instructions:

- ✓ Stand with your feet shoulder-width apart and make sure your knees are slightly bent.
- ✓ Place your hands on your hips to help maintain balance and stability.
- ✓ Take a deep breath and as you exhale, tilt your pelvis forward by tightening your abdominal muscles and tucking your tailbone under.

✓ Hold the pelvic tilt position for 5-10 seconds, focusing on contracting the muscles in your pelvic floor. You should feel a slight pulling sensation in your lower abdomen and pelvic region.

✓ Relax and release the pelvic tilt, returning to the starting position.

✓ Repeat the exercise for 10-15 repetitions, gradually increasing the number as you build strength and endurance.

Deep Squat

Deep squat is a great Kegel exercise for men to improve reproductive health.

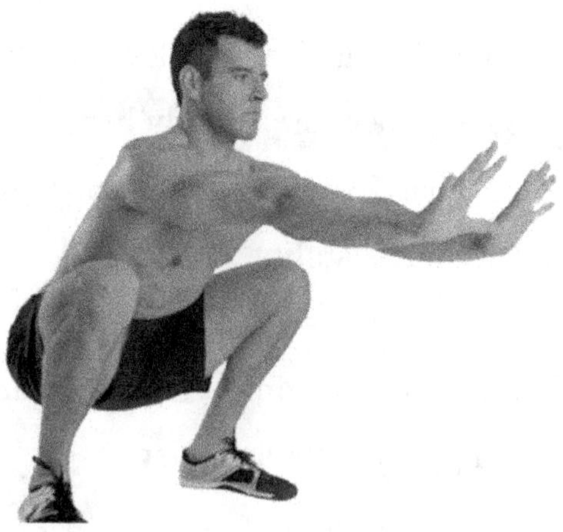

Instructions:

- ✓ Stand with your feet slightly wider than shoulder-width apart, with your toes pointed slightly outward.
- ✓ Lower your body down by bending your knees and hips, as if you are about to sit on a chair.
- ✓ Keep your back straight and chest up as you descend into the squat position. It's important to keep your weight on your heels and not on your toes.
- ✓ As you lower into the deep squat, engage your pelvic floor muscles by imagining pulling them upward as if trying to stop the flow of urine.
- ✓ Hold the deep squat position for 10-15 seconds, focusing on keeping the pelvic floor muscles engaged.
- ✓ Slowly rise back up to the starting position, keeping your pelvic floor engaged throughout the movement.
- ✓ Repeat the exercise for 10-15 repetitions, gradually increasing the number as you build strength and endurance.

Child's Pose

Child's pose is a yoga pose that can be modified to include Kegel exercises to improve reproductive health in men.

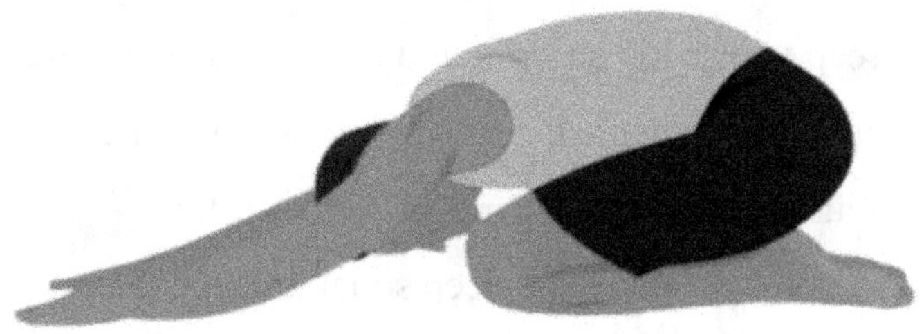

Instructions:

- ✓ Start by kneeling on the floor with your big toes together and your knees apart. Sit back on your heels.
- ✓ Slowly bend forward, lowering your torso towards the floor. Your forehead should rest on the ground, and your arms should be extended forward with your palms resting on the floor.
- ✓ Once in the child's pose position, take a deep breath, and as you exhale, engage your pelvic floor muscles by imagining pulling them upward as if trying to stop the flow of urine.

✓ Hold the engaged pelvic floor muscles for 10-15 seconds while maintaining the child's pose position.

✓ Relax and release the engagement of your pelvic floor muscles, allowing them to return to their resting state.

✓ Repeat the exercise for 10-15 repetitions, gradually increasing the number as you build strength and endurance.

The Butterfly Stretch

The Butterfly stretch is a simple and effective exercise that can be combined with Kegel exercises to improve reproductive health for men.

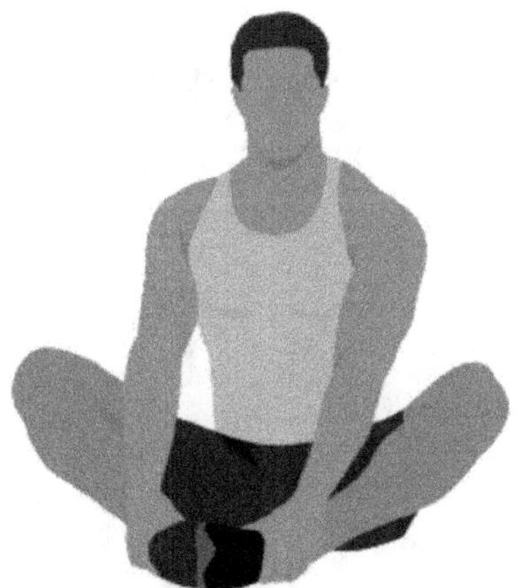

Instructions:

- ✓ Sit on the floor with your back straight and bring the soles of your feet together in front of your pelvis, allowing your knees to fall outward.
- ✓ Grasp your feet with your hands for support, and gently pull them closer to your body.
- ✓ Take a deep breath, and as you exhale, engage your pelvic floor muscles by imagining pulling them upward, as if trying to stop the flow of urine.
- ✓ Hold the engaged pelvic floor muscles for 10-15 seconds while maintaining the butterfly stretch position.
- ✓ Relax and release the engagement of your pelvic floor muscles, allowing them to return to their resting state.
- ✓ Repeat the exercise for 10-15 repetitions, gradually increasing the number as you build strength and endurance.

The Cobra Stretch

The Cobra stretch is a yoga pose that can be combined with Kegel exercises to improve reproductive health for men.

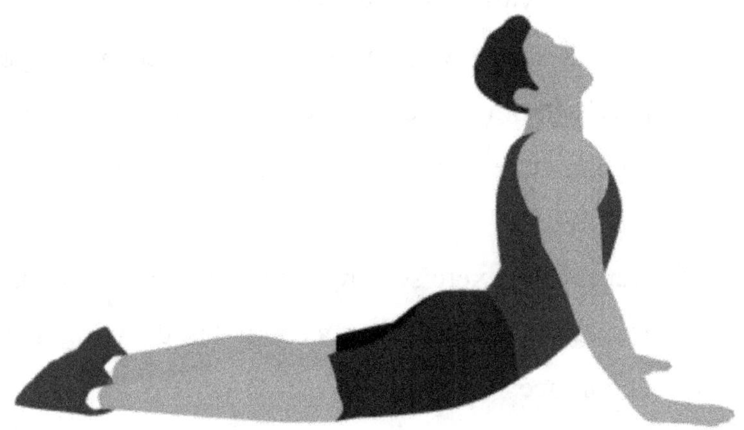

Instructions:

- ✓ Lie face down on the floor with your palms placed on the ground under your shoulders.
- ✓ Keep your legs extended behind you with the tops of your feet pressing into the floor.
- ✓ As you inhale, slowly straighten your arms to lift your chest off the ground, while keeping your pelvis and legs pressing into the floor.

- ✓ Engage your pelvic floor muscles by imagining pulling them upward as if trying to stop the flow of urine as you lift your chest.
- ✓ Hold the engaged pelvic floor muscles for 10-15 seconds while maintaining the cobra stretch position.
- ✓ Exhale and slowly release the engagement of your pelvic floor muscles, allowing them to return to their resting state as you lower your chest back down to the ground.
- ✓ Repeat the exercise for 10-15 repetitions, gradually increasing the number as you build strength and endurance.

The Lying Knee-To-Chest Stretch

The lying knee-to-chest stretch is a simple exercise that can be combined with Kegel exercises to improve reproductive health for men.

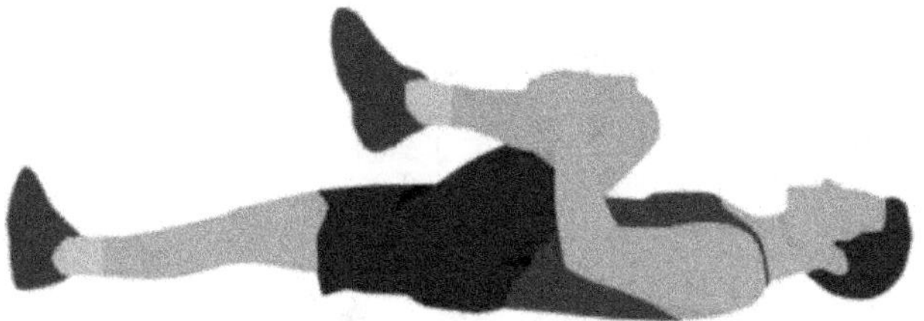

Instructions:

- ✓ Lie on your back on a comfortable surface such as a yoga mat or a bed.
- ✓ Bend your knees, keeping your feet flat on the surface and your arms resting alongside your body.
- ✓ Take a deep breath and as you exhale, bring one knee towards your chest using your hands to gently pull it closer.
- ✓ As you bring your knee to your chest, engage your pelvic floor muscles by imagining pulling them upward as if trying to stop the flow of urine.
- ✓ Hold the engaged pelvic floor muscles for 10-15 seconds while maintaining the knee-to-chest stretch position.
- ✓ Relax and release the engagement of your pelvic floor muscles, allowing them to return to their resting state as you lower your leg back down.

- ✓ Repeat the exercise with the opposite leg, and continue to alternate between legs for a balanced stretch.

The Pigeon Pose

The Pigeon Pose is a yoga stretch that may benefit men's reproductive health when combined with Kegel exercises.

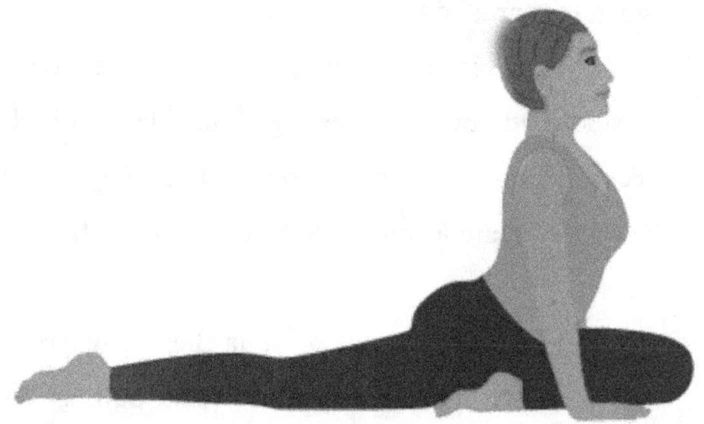

Instructions:

- ✓ Start in a tabletop position on the floor, with your hands and knees on the ground, and your wrists aligned with your shoulders.

- ✓ Lift your right knee off the floor and slide your right leg forward, bending your knee and bringing it toward your right wrist.

- ✓ Extend your left leg behind you, keeping your hips square to the front of the mat.

- ✓ Lower your hips towards the ground, feeling a stretch in the right hip and buttock.

- ✓ Take a deep breath, and as you exhale, engage your pelvic floor muscles by imagining pulling them upward, as if trying to stop the flow of urine.

- ✓ Hold the engaged pelvic floor muscles for 10-15 seconds while maintaining the pigeon pose position.

- ✓ Relax and release the engagement of your pelvic floor muscles, allowing them to return to their resting state.

- ✓ Repeat the exercise for 10-15 repetitions, gradually increasing the number as you build strength and endurance.

Kneeling Plank

Kneeling plank is a variation of the traditional plank exercise that targets the core muscles, including the pelvic floor muscles, which are important for reproductive health in men.

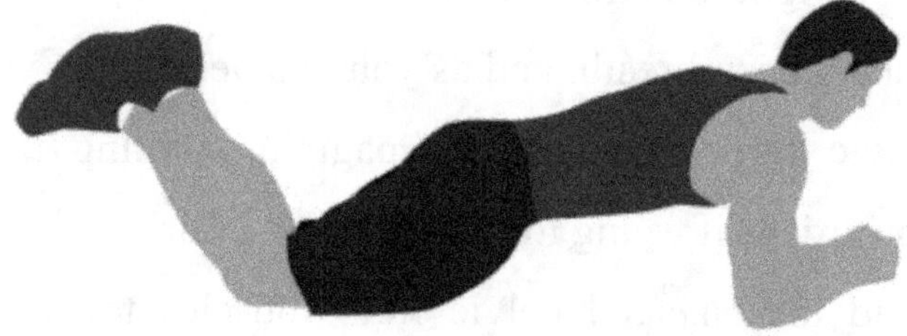

Instructions:

- ✓ Start by getting down on your hands and knees on a mat or soft surface. Ensure that your hands are directly under your shoulders and your knees are under your hips.

- ✓ Extend one leg straight out behind you and then the other, so that you are now in a plank position with your body forming a straight line from your head to your heels.

- ✓ Engage your core muscles and focus on squeezing your pelvic floor muscles as you hold the plank position.
- ✓ Hold the plank position for 10-30 seconds, breathing steadily throughout.
- ✓ As you get stronger, gradually increase the time you hold the plank position, aiming for 60 seconds or more.
- ✓ To complete the exercise, slowly lower your knees to the mat and rest for a moment before repeating the plank 2-3 more times.

The Leg Extension Plank

The Leg Extension Plank is a Kegel exercise that can help improve reproductive health for men by strengthening the pelvic floor muscles.

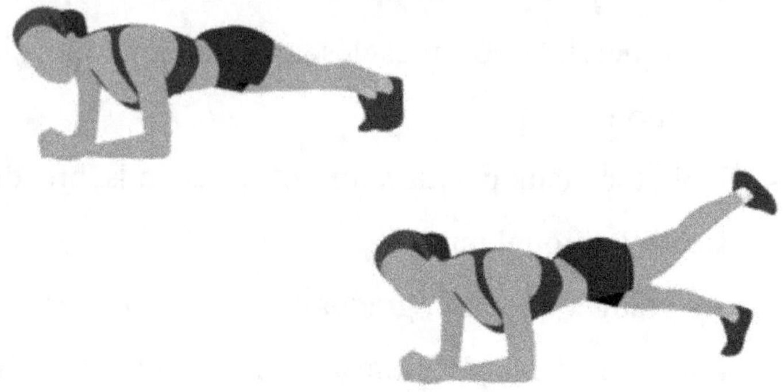

Instructions:

- ✓ Start by getting into a traditional plank position with your forearms on the ground, elbows directly under your shoulders, and legs extended behind you, forming a straight line from your head to your heels.

- ✓ Engage your core muscles, including the muscles of the pelvic floor, by pulling your navel towards your spine.

- ✓ Once you are in a stable plank position, slowly lift one leg off the ground, extending it straight behind you. Maintain as much stillness as possible throughout the remainder of your body.

- ✓ Hold the extended leg in the air for 5-10 seconds while maintaining the plank position and engaging your pelvic floor muscles.

- ✓ Slowly lower the extended leg back to the ground and switch to the other leg, repeating the same process.
- ✓ Aim to perform 8-10 leg extensions on each leg, alternating between sides, for a total of 16-20 extensions.

Reverse Plank

Reverse plank is a great exercise for strengthening the core, including the pelvic floor muscles, which are important for reproductive health in men.

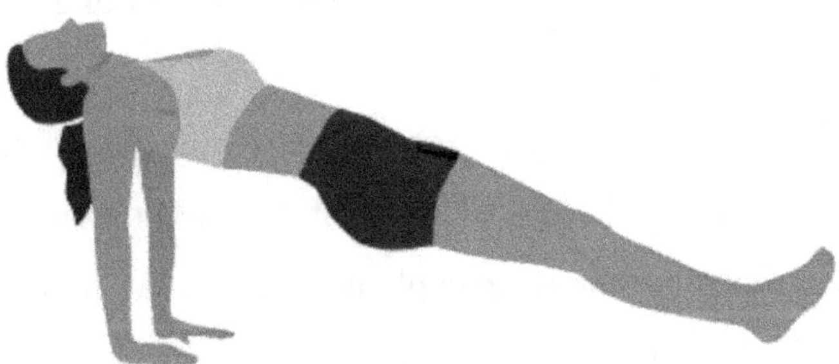

Instructions:

- ✓ Start by sitting on the floor with your legs extended in front of you and your hands placed on the floor slightly behind your hips, with your fingers pointing towards your feet.

✓ Press into your hands and lift your hips off the ground, creating a straight line from your head to your heels. Your shoulders should be directly above your wrists.

✓ Engage your core muscles and focus on squeezing your pelvic floor muscles as you hold the reverse plank position.

✓ Hold the reverse plank position for 10-30 seconds, breathing steadily throughout.

✓ As you get stronger, gradually increase the time you hold the reverse plank position, aiming for 60 seconds or more.

✓ To complete the exercise, slowly lower your hips back to the floor and rest for a moment before repeating the reverse plank for 2-3 more times.

The Bear Walk

The Bear Walk is a dynamic exercise that engages multiple muscle groups, including the core and pelvic floor muscles, and can contribute to improving reproductive health in men.

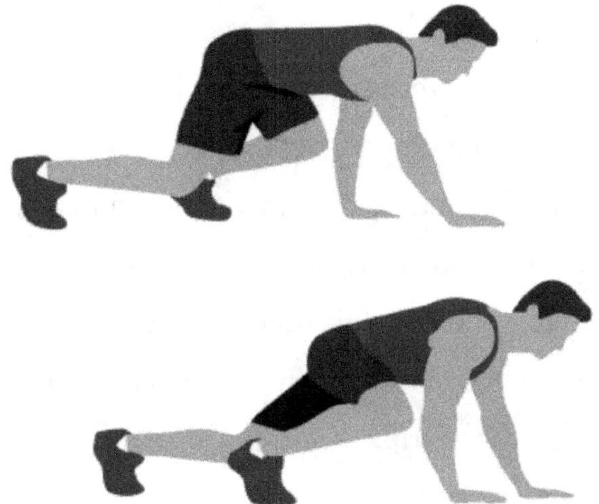

Instructions:

- ✓ Start in a tabletop position on the floor with your hands directly underneath your shoulders and your knees bent at a 90-degree angle beneath your hips.
- ✓ Lift your knees a few inches off the ground, keeping them bent at a 90-degree angle, so your weight is on your toes and hands.

✓ Engage your core muscles, including the muscles of the pelvic floor, by pulling your navel towards your spine.

✓ Begin to "walk" forward by moving your right hand and left foot forward simultaneously, followed by your left hand and right foot. This should create a crawling motion, similar to a bear.

✓ As you "walk" forward, focus on keeping your hips stable and your core engaged. The movement should be slow and controlled, with a focus on maintaining proper form and engaging the pelvic floor muscles.

✓ Continue walking in this bear crawl fashion for about 10-15 steps forward, then 10-15 steps backward, making a round trip.

Namaskar Asana Pose

Namaskar asana, also known as the prayer pose or "Anjali Mudra," is a common yoga posture that involves pressing the palms of the hands together in a gesture of reverence. While it's not a Kegel exercise in the traditional sense, yoga in general can help improve pelvic floor muscle strength and overall reproductive health in both men and women by improving circulation and reducing stress.

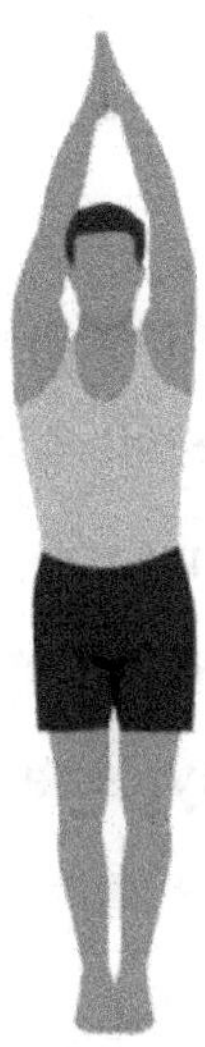

Instructions:

- ✓ Stand tall with your feet together or slightly apart, depending on your comfort. Maintain a straight spine and relaxed shoulders.
- ✓ Bring your hands together in front of your chest, with your palms pressed firmly against each other in a prayer-like gesture.
- ✓ Close your eyes, take a deep breath in, and then exhale slowly.

✓ While holding this position, focus on engaging your pelvic floor muscles. This can be done by gently contracting the muscles as if you're trying to stop the flow of urine. Hold this contraction for the duration of your breath.

✓ Repeat this process for 5-10 breaths, maintaining the engagement of the pelvic floor muscles and focusing on relaxation and mindfulness.

✓ Namaskar asana can be performed multiple times throughout the day, as a way to center and ground yourself, as well as engage the pelvic floor muscles.

The Crab Pose

The Crab Pose, also known as "Ardha Purvottanasana" in yoga, is a great way to engage the pelvic floor muscles and improve overall reproductive health in men.

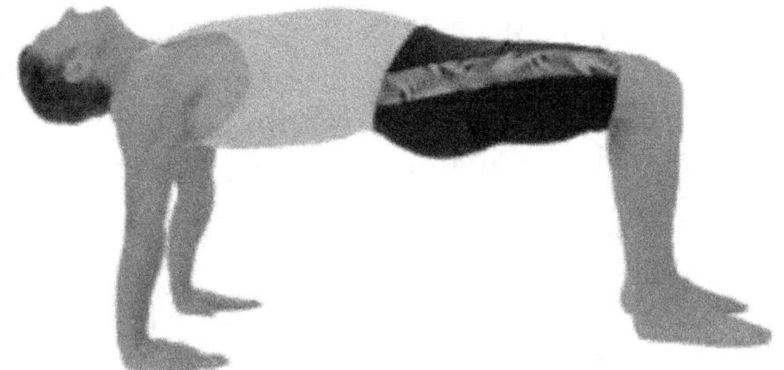

Instructions:

- ✓ Begin by sitting on the floor with your knees bent and feet flat on the ground about hip-width apart. Place your hands behind you with your fingers pointing toward your feet, and your palms flat on the ground.

- ✓ Press into your hands and feet, lifting your hips off the ground, and straightening your arms. Your body should form a reverse tabletop position with your hips lifted, chest open, and gaze facing forward.

- ✓ Engage your core muscles, including the muscles of the pelvic floor, by gently contracting the muscles as if you're trying to stop the flow of urine.

- ✓ Hold the Crab Pose for 15-30 seconds, focusing on maintaining steady breathing and the engagement of the pelvic floor muscles.
- ✓ Slowly lower your hips back to the ground to release the pose.
- ✓ Repeat the Crab Pose 3-5 times, with a focus on controlled movements and maintaining proper form.

Marching Feet

Although marching feet exercise does not directly target pelvic floor muscles, it can indirectly benefit reproductive health by engaging the core, which includes the pelvic floor muscles.

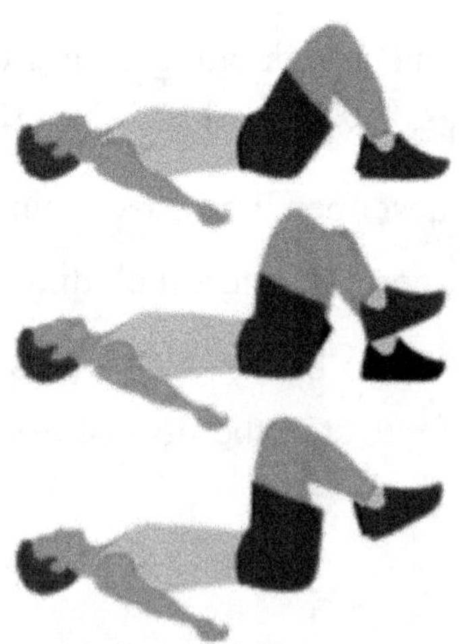

Instructions:

- ✓ Start by lying on your back with your arms by your sides and your knees bent.

- ✓ Engage your core muscles by drawing your navel towards your spine and pressing your lower back into the ground.

- ✓ Keeping your core engaged, slowly lift one foot off the ground, bringing your knee towards your chest.

- ✓ Lower the first foot back to the ground and then repeat the movement with the other foot, imitating a marching motion.

- ✓ Continue to alternate lifting each foot in a marching motion while maintaining engagement of the core muscles.

- ✓ Aim to perform 2-3 sets of 10-15 marches on each leg, focusing on controlled movements and steady breathing.

Glute March

Glute March is a Kegel exercise that targets the pelvic floor muscles, which can contribute to improving reproductive health in men. Here's a step-by-step guide on how to

perform the Glute March exercise along with recommendations for the duration and repetitions to improve reproductive health:

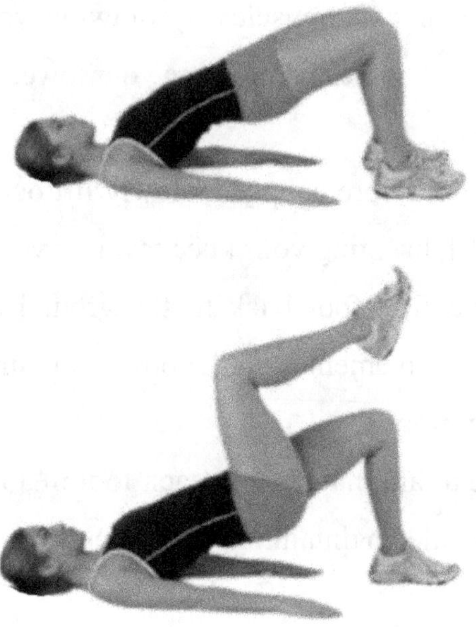

Instructions:

- ✓ Start by reclining on your back, knees bent, and feet flat on the floor. Maintain your arms at your sides.
- ✓ Engage your core muscles by gently drawing your navel towards your spine and pressing your lower back into the ground.
- ✓ Lift your hips off the ground, forming a bridge position, with your body weight supported by your

feet and shoulders. Your entire body should form a straight line from your shoulders to your knees.

- ✓ Engage your glutes and core to maintain the bridge position and prevent excessive arching in the lower back.

- ✓ With your hips lifted, slowly lift one foot off the ground, bringing your knee towards your chest, keeping your hips stable and level.

- ✓ Lower the first foot back to the ground and then repeat the movement with the other foot, imitating a marching motion while maintaining the bridge position.

- ✓ Continue to alternate lifting each foot in a marching motion while maintaining stable hips and a strong bridge position.

- ✓ Aim to perform 2-3 sets of 10-15 marches on each leg, focusing on controlled movements, stable hips, and engagement of the pelvic floor muscles.

Warrior II Pose

Warrior II pose, also known as Virabhadrasana II, is a foundational yoga pose that is excellent for strengthening the legs, stretching the hips, and improving overall stamina and concentration. It can also contribute to the improvement of reproductive health in men.

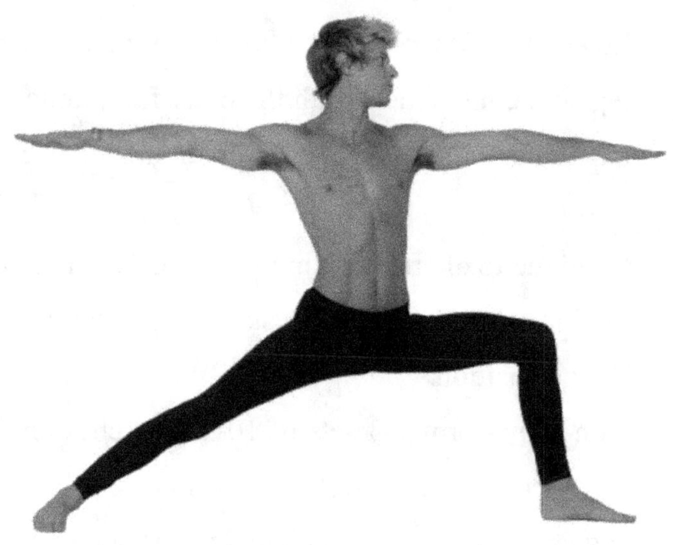

Instructions:

- ✓ Start standing at the top of your mat with your feet together.

- ✓ Step your left foot back about 3-4 feet, keeping your right foot facing forward and your left foot turned slightly inwards.
- ✓ Bend your right knee, making sure it stays directly over your ankle. Your left leg should be straight and strong.
- ✓ Extend your arms out to the sides at shoulder height, parallel to the floor.
- ✓ Keep your torso facing to the side, and gaze over your right hand.
- ✓ Relax your shoulders and reach through your fingertips.
- ✓ Hold the pose for 30 seconds to 1 minute, then switch to the other side.
- ✓ Repeat this process 10-15 times per set.
- ✓ Aim to complete 3-4 sets of these exercises per day.

Triangle Pose

Triangle pose, also known as Trikonasana, is a yoga pose that stretches and strengthens the entire body, including the legs, hips, spine, and shoulders. It is also known to aid in improving reproductive health in men.

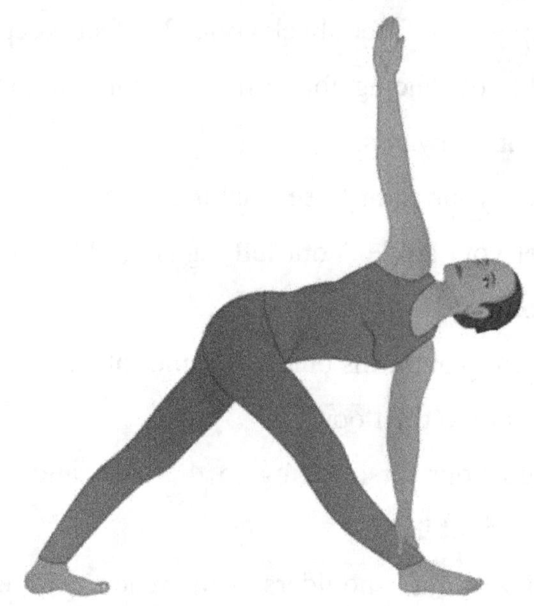

Instructions:

- ✓ Start standing at the top of your mat with your feet about 3-4 feet apart.

- ✓ Turn your right foot out ninety (90) degrees and your left foot in about forty-five (45) degrees.

- ✓ Extend your arms out to the side at shoulder height, and reach as far as you can to the right, hinging at your hips.

- ✓ Lower your right hand down to your right shin, ankle, or the floor (depending on your flexibility), and extend your left arm straight up towards the ceiling.

✓ Keep your chest and hips open, and avoid collapsing into the right side of your body.

✓ Keep your gaze either straight ahead or up at your left hand.

✓ Hold the pose for 30 seconds to 1 minute, then come back up to standing and repeat on the other side.

Sumo Squats

Sumo squats are a type of squat that target the inner thighs, glutes, and hamstrings. It can be beneficial for improving reproductive health in men due to the engagement of the pelvic floor muscles during the exercise.

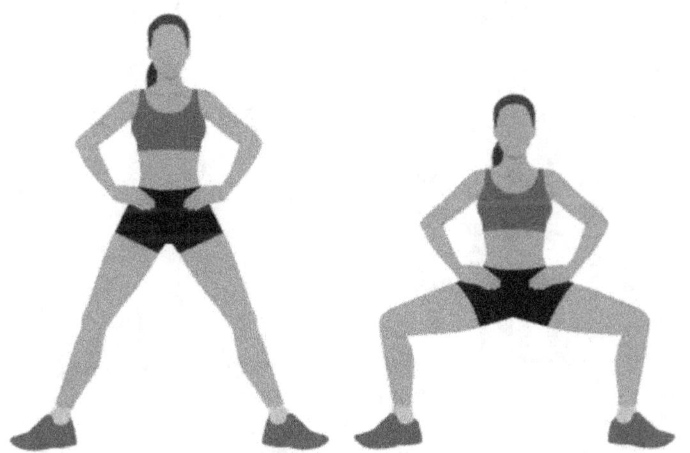

Instructions:

- ✓ Stand with your feet wider than hip-width apart, with your toes pointed slightly outward.
- ✓ Keep your back straight, chest up, and shoulders down.
- ✓ Engage your core muscles to stabilize your torso.
- ✓ Lower your body down by bending at the knees and hips, as if you are going to sit back into a chair.
- ✓ Aim to lower your hips until your thighs are parallel to the ground. Maintain proper knee-to-toe alignment.
- ✓ Push through your heels to return to the starting position, squeezing your glutes at the top.
- ✓ Repeat for 10-15 repetitions, for 2-3 sets.

CONCLUSION

The practice of Kegel exercises offers men a transformative pathway to regain control over their reproductive health and sexual wellness. By dedicating time and effort to these targeted exercises, men have the opportunity to enhance their fertility, address concerns related to premature ejaculation, and tackle issues of erectile dysfunction. With consistent commitment, men can unlock the potential to improve their endurance, confidence, and overall sexual satisfaction. The journey to reclaiming vitality and vigor begins with the simple yet impactful steps of Kegel exercises. Embrace this empowering practice, and step into a future of renewed virility and sexual fulfillment.

www.ingramcontent.com/pod-product-compliance
Lightning Source LLC
Chambersburg PA
CBHW060915130726
48001CB00006B/2257